I0116522

Dethroning the American Medical System

Dethroning the American Medical System

Taking Personal Responsibility For Your Healthcare

by

Marie Rosalind Churchill

Dethroning the American Medical System
Copyright 2014 by Marie Rosalind Churchill

Printed and bound in the United States of America.   All rights reserved. No part of this book may be reproduced in any form or by electronic or mechanical means including information storage and retrieval systems without permission in writing from the publisher, Brief quotes as specified in United States Copyright Act of 1976 as currently revised are excepted.

Unless otherwise indicated, all scripture references/quotations are taken from the authorized King James Version of the Bible used by permission.

Cover Design © 2014

All Rights Reserved

Protected by United States and International copyright laws as currently revised.

Note: In this publication, the word "he" has been used rather than he/she for a doctor of either gender. "She" has been used rather than she/he for a nurse of either gender. These choices were made to eliminate confusion, realizing that persons of either gender occupy roles as nurses and doctors.

educationalresource@tipstoahealthieryou.info

First Edition 2014 trade paperback

ISBN-10: 0989473546
ISBN-13:9780989473545

DEDICATION

This book is dedicated to my wonderful and loving parents, and to my faithful friend—and lifelong spouse.

Special thanks to my writing mentor and to my writing groupies. In addition, I also want to thank my faithful friend for her persistent encouragement and to all who were the audience for my ideas as they became this book.

CONTENTS

Information offered here is presented to encourage personal responsibility for health care. We do not offer medical diagnosis, mental or physical, and are not a substitute for health care. No responsibility is assumed on the part of the author, publishers or distributors of this book for your personal choices in health care.

PREFACE

Have you wanted to reduce the medical expenses incurred by your family? Maybe you want to avoid that feeling of being a powerless victim of the medical system? Perhaps you have health questions and need an expert to help you? Then you are the person for whom this book is written.

Although a medical doctor is an authority in the field of medicine, he is not an authority about *you*. He is a professional, hired to do a job for you, just as you would hire a plumber or car mechanic or some other specifically trained professional.

Some people may be convinced that a doctor is responsible for their body's health—not so—the doctor is only an agent to help steer <u>you</u> in the right direction.

A physician may prescribe a special diet or medication for you, but it is your responsibility to apply the diet or take the prescription according to the instructions. Once you accept this, you can begin learning to care for your own health.

You Are A Masterpiece

No one on earth looks exactly like you, even if you have an identical twin. You are beautiful and unique:

- Your hair.
- Your freckles.
- Your abilities.
- Your size.

You are The Creator's masterpiece sent to the rest of the world. As a masterpiece you require proper care.

It is important to invest time learning to distinguish the difference between our inherent, physical traits and signs of something physically wrong or going wrong in our bodies.

As an art museum curator is able to distinguish between character changes (inherent traits) in a painting, and actual damage beginning in an art piece, we should be able to recognize those changes in our body.

Performing a weekly overview of your masterpiece is one of the best ways to observe the condition of your body and to determine when closer examination is needed. Take it out of the frame, so to speak. Stand in front of a full length **glass** mirror in your birthday suit, or as some people say, "naked as the day you were born." Plastic mirrors reflect a warped view which will not allow a true assessment of you; *the masterpiece.*

You are not comparing yourself with how you want to be or how somebody else is. You are simply looking at your physical condition—muscle tone, fat deposits, and characteristics such as freckles, varicose veins, warts, and even rashes. Do this once a week for a few months so that you know what your masterpiece looks like. Get used to looking at you!

As you observe yourself week after week, you will be able to notice tiny changes that have occurred during the month—a mole may be getting larger/smaller—rashes may resolve, love handles may increase or shrink.

In addition to observing, don't be afraid to touch yourself, checking for changes in the texture of your skin or body parts.

The important thing is to learn what is normal for you and then check for changes from <u>that</u> normal. Look for symmetry. Posture should be equal on both sides of your body. Shoulders and hips should be about even as should breasts if you are a woman. Your navel should be centered approximately at your natural waistline.

Remember to thank your Maker for creating you the way you are, no matter what you think you should look like. The characteristics that you complain about may be the very things that God considers beautiful and unique about you.

Another thing to consider when observing yourself is the overall shape of your body. The common shape for a healthy person of any age would be the tower shape where it appears one part is set right on top of another— erect and slim. Any other shape may indicate the beginning of internal problems.

Growing a belly is not healthy-unless you are pregnant. It means that metabolism has slowed and internal organs have begun building up fat. A fatty organ is not operating at top efficiency and will most likely break down.

Some people find that they have difficulty getting around easily, perhaps, because of a previous surgery or just sitting too much. This should not be ignored.

Rather, an appointment should be made with a physical therapist to develop a routine for strengthening and mobilizing your body. You may need a prescription from a medical doctor if you wish your insurance to pay for this service.

Putting exercise on your weekly schedule will do much to promote long healthy life and vitality as will eating things which are actually food, rather than palatable plastics which often are packaged as food.

Learn all you can about your body to help yourself stay healthy and strong. Why wait until there is pain, or perhaps a lump, before caring about the condition of your masterpiece? Study up on anything that does not appear to be healthy. Ask questions about anything that concerns you.

It may be tempting to decorate the outside of your body with clothes, makeup, and jewelry in an attempt to ignore or camouflage its needs. Please realize that decorations won't fix anything and in fact may cover serious problems, allowing them to become life threatening.

Some people live as though their bodies are their own to abuse. They do not think about learning to eat well or exercising to strengthen their physical frames. Do you think we would have the Mona Lisa or the statue of David or other masterpieces if museums were as thoughtless with the valuable art in their care?

In a museum, the atmosphere is carefully controlled for the good of the artwork. Temperature, humidity and light levels are all monitored and automatically adjusted to prevent unnecessary aging. Wouldn't it be wise to use preventative care in the management of <u>your</u> masterpiece?

The fact is, you ARE the expert about yourself. It may surprise you to know that your doctor relies on <u>your</u> observation of <u>yourself</u> to know what is wrong with you.

You may have gone to a doctor only to

have him ask you a series of questions:
- Why did you come in here today?
- What seems to be the problem?

You tell him why you have come in and he asks you more questions:
- How long have you had that?
- Has it changed?
- Is this usual for you?

A physician relies on you to work with him to diagnose a condition and then he decides on the course of treatment.

Change Should Be Gradual

As you observe yourself weekly, watch for signs of change. Changes in your body should be extremely gradual, not sudden. Anytime something changes in a way that does not look right to you, ask about it.

In general, younger people tend to develop conditions of deficiency or excess while people 50 and older tend to develop wearing-out conditions. How we take care of our masterpiece when we are young will determine what will happen when we are older. A good example of this would be a former football player who sustained a knee injury during his athletic career which affects the way he walks today.

Gradual change may mean that your masterpiece is aging. Signs of aging mean you are becoming more valuable. Don't buy into the lie that you won't be valuable when you are old. God values experience just as a museum values antiques. The difference between an antique and a piece of old junk is the care taken of the piece as it aged.

Who Do You Ask?

Where do you start when you have questions about your body? Who do you talk with?

My suggestion would be to look around in your church congregation for a nurse, preferably a registered nurse trained at the Bachelor level. Nurses are trained to look at the entire body as a whole and have experience working in the medical field. They can often give you a nursing diagnosis[1] which is based on your body's needs, and may include general treatments you can do yourself.

---

[1]A nursing diagnosis is based on your own bodily responses to a condition change.

Nurses are usually kind people who are willing to take some time to help you. Hospital nurses are preferable to office nurses, because nurses in hospitals make many of the decisions for patient care, while nurses in doctor's offices follow orders rather than make independent decisions.

If, however, you talk with a nurse who is grumpy, just go find another one to talk with. The grumpy nurse may be working too many hours or be under some personal stress and can use your kindness.

If you are unable to find a nurse to work with, you may consult with our nurses[2]

---

[2] See contact us page in the appendix

When first making arrangements with a nurse or other educational partner, ask if he/she prefers you to make an appointment. Explain that you want to ask a short question or two. Do not expect the nurse to spend hours examining your entire medical history. Think through your question so that you know what you want to ask. For example, "Does this mole look normal?"

You are not looking for cheap medical care. Your purpose is to find an educational partner who will be able to help you determine what is normal and usual for your body so that you may begin to recognize potential problems.

Others who could probably answer questions for you would be:

- A nutritionist, (not a dietician who is trained to do hospital menus.
- A physical therapist or perhaps even a massage therapist.

You are looking for education, not a diagnosis.

While in this research phase, you should also evaluate prescriptions you are currently taking. Ask yourself:

- Why am I taking this?
- What are the side effects?
- What changes have occurred in my body as a result of taking this medication?

You could buy a nurses' drug text for

reference which will help you gather the information you need[3]. Pay attention to the sections titled "contraindications." Online references may not be up-to-date, but, are certainly better than nothing.

If you have any questions about medications or their impact on your body ask a pharmacist rather than your doctor. A pharmacist may also be able to suggest substitutes for particular medications, if you are experiencing annoying or dangerous side effects.

After talking with the pharmacist, go back and talk with your doctor about the suggestions you received from the

---

[3] Nurse's Drug Handbooks are based not on the action of the drug but the person's response to them. Davis, Lippincott and many others may be available at your local library. Not the same as the Physician's Drug Reference.

pharmacist. The relationship between pharmacists and doctors is rather complicated—a synergistic one rather than a partnership. Pharmacists cannot prescribe medications and doctors cannot dispense medications except prepackaged samples.

People sometimes take their body to the doctor and basically turn it over, like taking a car in for repair. Haven't you heard of malpractice? Doctors are human and **can** make mistakes. Any mistakes <u>they</u> make are <u>yours</u> to bear.

After assuring yourself that there is indeed a reason to be seen by a health professional, pick out an office or an individual and schedule a visit to introduce yourself, so you and the doctor can get to know each other. You will want to check out the heart attitudes of those who will help you. Take the time to schedule an introductory consultation first, to meet with the provider as a person, rather than as a professional.

"Get to know you," consultations with doctors or other health practitioners are often free. Call the office and ask. Since you are there to meet the provider, not to get free advice. Keep your questions general.

Philosophy and Training
Of
Physicians

Don't allow yourself to be over-whelmed by the title "Doctor". There are many schools of training for physicians, each reflect differences in philosophy and treatments.

The most common doctor in practice today is the allopathic or medically trained physician[4]. Usually allopathic doctors diagnose by tests such as blood tests and other invasive procedures. They prescribe medicines which are chemical in nature, although some may have an herbal extract in the compilation. These doctors will have MD after their name.

Many medical doctors are also trained in law. Because of this, the doctor may do extra tests to rule out mistakes, which, of course, raises the cost to

[4] For further information-see definition pages in appendix

you. These extra tests may be more to protect the doctor from future lawsuits than for ruling out diseases.

Other types of doctors may include chiropractic, naturopathic, herbalist, homeopathic, or vitalist. These doctors practice in specialties which do not usually use chemical medications.

Some may send you to a health or natural food store and others may give you herbal medications or herbal extracts (called tinctures).

In the initial interview it would be wise to ask what kind of treatments might be used. Some doctors call their treatments modalities.

Treatments used by alternative

practitioners, or therapists, will vary widely. Most will use non-invasive diagnostic tests and treatments since they do not break the "skin barrier." With very few exceptions, "breaking the skin barrier" is legally limited to medical professionals.

Medical professionals, including chiropractors, are considered "mainstream." Most others would be considered "alternative" because they are different from the mainstream.

I would encourage you to search for a practitioner educated in looking at the entire body as a whole. Perhaps you could find an older chiropractor or a naturopath. By older, I mean one that has been in practice for longer than 20 years. If you find a naturopath, ask what kind of tests would likely be ordered. If they order blood work and other lab tests, they are medically trained and the total costs to you would be higher than for a traditionally trained naturopath, using herbs and other non-medical treatments.

Doctors are trained to concentrate on only one problem at a time. Therefore, if you are concerned about a wart you have been treating at home with no success and go to the doctor about another condition, they probably will tell you to make a separate appointment for the wart. This is how they are trained to build their practice.

Nurse practitioners are another group

not yet mentioned. These are nurses who have additional training in the medical field, further licensed by the nursing board to make medical diagnoses and prescribe chemical medications.

Being a nurse practitioner means that although they are practicing in the medical field, they still are viewing the body as a whole. This is important because we are whole people, not a bunch of individual parts stuck together.

Physician assistants are actually doctors who have been trained to assist other doctors. The assistant may see some of the doctor's clients, diagnose and prescribe, but must have the doctor co-sign his records. This does not mean these individuals are less capable or safe. It is simply a legal distinction of the licensing board for physicians.

No matter whom you choose for your health practitioner, schedule a get-to-know-you consultation and then follow that up with research. Ask the practitioner about his/her licensing and accreditation. It would be acceptable to ask for contact information so that you will understand the licensing agency's philosophy.

A medical doctor may give you an odd reaction at this point. Give him/her the benefit of the doubt. Medical schools teach doctors to protect their own, and they may adopt a defensive attitude if you ask for more information. Be polite. Let the doctor know that you feel responsible to know more about a person who will help *You* make crucial decisions for your life.

It is important to get correct information. Medical doctors are somewhat like salesmen. They have to adopt a manner which elicits confidence especially when they suggest treatments that are painful or distasteful. Good health is not about obeying the doctor, rather it is about making healthy personal choices.

One of the purposes of the get-to-know-you appointment is to understand the doctors philosophy. If you have a difference in opinion about treatments you need to feel confident that your doctor will not be mad at you for your choice. It is not appropriate to feel scolded or worried about what your doctor will think of your health care decisions.

Ask questions! An honest answer will be helpful to you—while a situation in which a practitioner avoids answering you, will not. Ask the Heavenly Father to help you. He has sent the Holy Spirit to guide you into all truth [5].

Many doctors currently in training are working toward becoming a specialist.

---

[5] See appendix John 16:15

I would suggest you try to find a general practitioner. I especially like to work with older doctors who have been in general practice for years. Their experience is valuable. They are not usually anxious to operate or give unneeded prescriptions and are more willing to take the time to educate you. If they think that specialized tests are needed, they may send you to a specialist.

Specialists do tend to order more tests than general practitioners, which will mean additional costs for you. In addition, they tend to perform more surgeries. Just because you hear something from a specialist does not mean that you should cease doing your own research.

Make Good Healthcare Decisions

Research should not be performed as a social activity, such as talking with friends, Facebook, or discussion group threads. Use a good medical dictionary such as Taber's[6] along with the Merck Manual, a handbook developed by a pharmaceutical company to help standardize medical diagnosis and prescribing[7]. It is updated frequently and will list most diseases and conditions, currently accepted treatments, medications prescribed, and prognosis.

Again, just because you read

---

[6] Taber's Cyclopedic Medical Dictionary- F.A. Davis co Philadelphia © 2013 in the 22nd edition.

[7] Merck manuals can be purchased online at www.merckmanuals.com For more information about the Merck Manual see the appendix.

something in the Merck Manual does not mean that you must immediately decide to follow that advice. If something does not seem the best choice for you, check it out.

Every family would do well to have access to a copy of a medical dictionary and a Merck Manual. These can be purchased online[8]. You may find that your local library has a current copy. When your practitioner says you have XYZ and you must do a certain thing or you will die, Do not just accept this as the truth. It may be or it may not be. *Listen to your doctor and take very careful notes—then check it out.*

---

[8] Merck manuals can be purchased online at www.merckmanuals.com. For more information about the Merck Manual see the appendix

Look everything up in the Merck manual, including the usual treatments and medications recommended. After you have the information you need concerning any diagnosis or condition, treatment, test, or medication that is suggested for you, talk with your family and pray about it before making your decision.

It is never appropriate to be rushed into surgery or radical tests without time to consult with your family and think about it. This would be especially true when the procedure or treatment carries life-changing implications.

Informed Consent

Informed Consent is a very important aspect of medical care. All practitioners should be using this for any test, treatment, or medication offered. This information is required—do not let it be skipped! Here is the information they should be discussing with you:

Diagnosis: Disease you may have—explained in everyday terms

Prognosis: What to expect—how long the diagnoses condition is expected to last.

Usual treatment options: What the doctor is offering you.

Alternatives available: You may have to research these yourself

Side effects of treatments or medication: The doctor may not know without looking these up, but they may be drastic.

<u>Other possible physical or emotional reactions</u>: Clear explanations should be given of what they are proposing and why they think this is the best choice for you.

The medical office should have printed information with pictures to help you understand. If the doctor does not present this information, ask for it.

Always pay attention to what your gut is saying. God promises He will never leave us or forsake us and He also promises to send us His Spirit to teach us and to guide us.

Our hearts should always be at peace

with our decisions. When they are not—we need to rethink our current life decisions.

****

I have known people who have been fired by the medical doctor they were seeing because they would not do everything he told them to do. Yes, your doctor can actually fire you as a client. However, regretting a surgery you didn't want to have or suffering major complications as a result for the rest of your life can be much more difficult than putting up with a paternalistic doctor.

You can always change doctors if your provider is getting an attitude, but you cannot change bodies. Do the research. Ask questions. Pray for wisdom and help.

I would like to make one last comment concerning medical care. In the case of trauma: severe car accident, gunshot wound, or accidental dismemberment, the medical doctor would be the only expert to use. They have the equipment and the surgical experience and can save lives where some alternative methods of healing would not be fast enough or invasive enough.

In the case of such trauma, go to the hospital or to an allopathic physician immediately and ask questions later.

Medically Induced Disease

We have not yet covered the subject of iatrogenic disease or nosocomial infection. According to Taber's Medical

Dictionary, an iatrogenic disease is any injury or illness that occurs as a result of medical care[9].

A nosocomial infection is an infection acquired in-hospital, nursing home, or other health care setting. Taber's lists numerous infections that can be obtained simply by being in the hospital[10]. Over two million nosocomial infections occur in the U.S. annually. Antibiotic-resistant organisms such as clostridium-difficile, Enterobacter, Pseudomonas, staphylococci, enterococci, and various fungi often are responsible for the infectious outbreaks that result.

---

[9] (p1239)Taber's Cyclopedic Medical Dictionary,22nd edition, F.A. Davis Co, Philadelphia © 2013
[10] http://www.tabers.com/tabersonline

Immunizations

Because I am writing this book to help you learn about working with the health care system, we should talk about immunizations.

I personally believe that vaccinations cripple the immune system. This happens because the immune system is distracted from the job it should be doing, causing it to become overwhelmed with the new task and unable to fight correctly.

I have observed that flu and pneumonia vaccinations are given during the winter season when people often succumb after taking the immunization, rather than during the warmer weather when most people are healthier.

Rather than simply developing a healthy immunity, many people actually come down with some variant of the illness. Every year many people get so sick they have to have an antibiotic to get over it. Some end up in the hospital, and some even die.

Unfortunately many of these are children, or older people, the very group that is targeted for immunization!

It appears that the whole system is carried out in a manner that develops the least success in obtaining immunity, rather than the most success.

I have also noticed that poorer communities offer vaccinations in the fall or winter, whereas the more wealthy communities offer their shots in the late summer. This makes an interesting comparison to think about.

Let's ask ourselves, is it the pharmaceutical companies, or the weather, which <u>create</u> the flu season?

Since the pharmaceutical laboratory cannot accurately predict the future, they cannot know what species will hit the nation, unless they are the ones who <u>created</u> it.

Anyone who experiences adverse effects from vaccinations or immunizations should report the matter immediately to the medical professional who administered the injection and to the website set up to register them[11].

H.I.P.P.A.

Before we go any further, we should discuss the <u>H</u>ealth <u>I</u>nsurance <u>P</u>ortability and <u>P</u>rivacy <u>A</u>ct.

The general public understands that HIPPA protects their privacy. However, if you actually read the document you are signing you will see that you agree to allow the doctor/dentist to share your information with any one of hundreds of governmental agencies and insurance companies, without your further consent.

---

[11]Parents may file their own report on vaccination complications at (800) 822-7967 For more information go to www.uaers.hhs.gov

Before this "privacy act" the doctor could not share your information with anyone, not even the insurance company. Not even with you.

Now it seems that not only is your information available to you, but to everyone else who thinks they have a right to it. Your dentist, optometrist and physician all share the same information on one huge database. It makes me wonder who else has access to this information, and how secure is this privacy.

*Why did it take legislation to bring this into being, if it really is **only** for medical providers?*

My Personal Preferences

Many people have asked me what kind of doctor would I see if I needed medical care. My personal choice would be a nurse-practitioner. I have also gone to an urgent care clinic, on occasion—simply to save time. This would be, however, more expensive than an office visit.

Chemical medications would be my <u>last</u> choice in treatments, since they have a tendency to rearrange the symptoms, and the problem will usually show up somewhere else later. In addition, they have many side effects and should be considered poison unless we absolutely need them.

For myself, I use a variety of over-the-counter herbal remedies and only resort to prescription medication if the herbal treatments have not succeeded in a reasonable amount of time.

Healthcare in Pregnancy And Birth

Two separate kinds of care for women in the healthy state of pregnancy would be medical care and midwifery care. Generally, midwifery care costs less and is more educational.

Midwives are taught to give care for women having normal pregnancies which would be ninety percent of all pregnancies, and obstetricians are trained to treat the remaining ten percent.

In America, we seem to have this out of balance: 90% of the births happen with obstetricians and midwives care for the remaining 10%.

Both midwives and physicians will provide good care, but more interventions and tests will occur while in the care of a doctor. If you prefer a doctor, search for a general practitioner rather than an obstetrician so you can avoid extra tests which may put baby in jeopardy, and would probably cost more.

A general practitioner may also refer you to an obstetrician if complications arise. So, if you are at a higher risk you may not have much choice in where you give birth or who will assist you.

Risk is a statistical way of looking at potential health problems, as indicated by medical and obstetrical history.

Next, think about where you want to give birth. Hospitals are common but have the highest rate of infections for moms and babies. Other places to consider would be home birth or an out-of-hospital birth center. Statistics tell us that home is the safest place to give birth, both for mothers and infants.

If you are pregnant for the first time and don't know where to start, find a midwife and ask a lot of questions. At least you will get a lot of information that could be useful later.

Sometimes a person may be considered high-risk in one pregnancy but not in the next, such as a woman carrying a breech baby.

Questions you could ask a midwife or doctor:

- What kind of training have you had?
- How many babies have you delivered?
- Tell me about your philosophy of birth.
- Have you ever lost a baby or a mom?
- Have any mothers contracted an infection while under your care?
- What are your arrangements with a pediatrician?

If you want a midwife and have been unable to locate one contact us for a referral website.

Relieving Minor Upsets

Before we close, I would suggest some research ideas for relieving minor upsets:

White Oak Bark: reputed to heal hemorrhoids, shrink tissues and strengthen blood vessels.

Valerian Root: natural sedative and sleep-aid.

Ginger Root: neutralizes acids and toxins in the digestive tract relieving gas and bloating.

Pau D'Arco: *a bitter tree bark with properties as an* antifungal, anti-viral and anti-inflammatory.

Charcoal powder: absorbs gas and bacteria in the intestinal tract—should be taken between meals.

Capsules of Cranberry powder: assist in maintaining acid levels in the urine preventing some infections.

Slippery Elm Bark: soothes minor bowel problems and constipation.

Nettle: relieves allergies and hay fever.

****

Our Father is a very great and masterful creator. He only makes good things and **<u>YOU</u>** are one.

He loves you very much. Even before you have been formally introduced He has sent you His love letter: the Holy Bible[12] with instructions for living.

****

---

[12] See appendix-love letter

Clearing Up the Details

Staying healthy is about making good personal choices.

- Eating healthy foods.
- Drinking enough pure water.
- Keeping your bowels regular.
- Exercise consistently.
- Don't overeat
  - thereby overwhelming the liver and gall bladder.
- Get enough sleep.
- Set aside one day per week for rest and recuperation.

Appendix 1
The Spiritual Factor

Sometimes people are in a rush to get
going and do things for God.
He is more interested in spending time
with you than <u>watching</u> you minister
for Him.

* * *

Spend at least five minutes every day
telling your heavenly Father your
concerns. Ask Him for help regarding
your daily life and choices. Ask him to
deal with them. He loves to talk with
you. Do it daily.

Appendix 2
Definitions

Allopathic Medicine: Conventional medical treatment of diagnosing symptoms. Uses substances or techniques to oppress or suppress symptoms. Also termed western medicine or evidence-based medicine and sometimes also known as modern medicine.

A Second Definition: The system of medical practice by use of remedies or drugs or surgery producing effects different from or incompatible with those produced by disease being treated.

Allopathic Medicine was named by

Samuel Hahnemann in 1810, to distinguish it from Homeopathy which he practiced.

Holistic: a Greek word meaning all, whole , entire, total.

Wholistic Medicine: A striving on the part of medicine to balance body, mind and spirit in order to allow healing to occur naturally.

Holistic/Wholistic: are used inter-changeably to describe treatment which involves every aspect of a human life. Both are considered a specialty of practice in addition to being a lens with which to view the patient and their needs.

Nursing: Nurses examine the human

response to actual or potential health challenges. In addition nurses make "care plans" which assist them and the nursing care team in focusing treatments which make changes to head the patient back to health.

Nurses are taught to examine the entire life and circumstances of an individual to determine care needs. Not only the area of physical illness, but the organs and systems of the body involved, plus, the emotional, physical, mental and spiritual relationships involving the person.

In addition, nurses view the financial, religious, friendships, significant family relationships, hobbies, relaxation, employment, vocation, and many other factors which make up each individual they care for. This is a great deal more than caring for a limited disease in one part of the body.

Appendix 3
Historical Information

You may wonder, how did the health care system become so complicated?

In the 18th and 19th centuries, every home had at least one family member knowledgeable and skilled in the use of herbs and healing agents. Some people who were especially skilled in healing opened their homes as hospitals and sanitariums.[13] There was not an officially accepted system of doctoring—schools of medicine were many and varied.

During this period, allopathic medicine

---

[13] Jethro Kloss, *Back to Eden*, Promise Kloss Moffett *"Memoirs of His Daughter"* (Twin Lakes, WI, Lotus Preess 2005,xiv

consisted of bloodletting and purging with poisonous plants and metals, such as mercury. This was a dark chapter in health care, with many "patients" dying of the cure, rather than the disease.

In the early 1900s, several wealthy groups put their political and financial support behind the allopathic schools of medicine. In addition, they financially supported the newly developing pharmaceutical laboratories.

To make a long story short, most of the other schools of healing went out of business and allopathic schools and pharmacies emerged as the only focus of medicine in America.

Since families ate healthier with fewer processed foods available and fewer chemical additives in foods, people tended to die of old age rather than degenerative diseases. In addition, people exercised more as part of daily living.

There was not much need for the new doctors. In fact, to make a living, most doctors in the early 1900s went house to house trying to drum up business. This introduced the "house call".

The value of the new allopathic doctors was their ability in trauma cases, which is still the case today.[14]

---

[14] Section taken from Green Pharmacy-The History and Evolution of Western Herbal Medicine

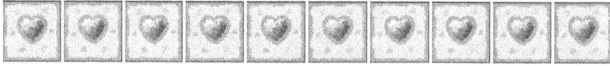

GOD'S LOVE LETTER

For God so loved the world that He gave His only begotten Son, that whosoever believeth in Him should not perish but have everlasting life.

For God sent not His Son into the world to condemn the world; but that the world through Him might be saved.

John 3:16-17

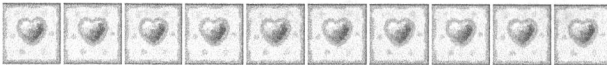

REFERENCES

1: For God so loved the world that He gave His only begotten Son, that whosoever believeth in Him should not perish but have everlasting life. For God sent not His Son into the world to condemn the world; but that the world through Him might be saved [John 3:16-17].

2:...Know ye not that your body is the temple of the Holy Ghost which is in you, which you have of God, and ye are not your own? For ye are bought with a price: therefore glorify God in your body, and in your spirit, which are God's [1 Corinthians 6:19-20].

3: Ask the Father to guide you. *He has sent you the Holy Spirit to guide you into all truth* [John 16:13a].

4: "A good man out of the good treasure of his heart bringeth forth that which is good; and an evil man out of the evil treasure of his heart bringeth forth that which is evil: for out of the abundance of the heart his mouth speaketh" Luke 6:45.

About the Author

The author uses her wide variety of training to educate the public, encouraging individuals to make life-long personal choices toward optimum health. Her views on health cover the medical spectrum and extend to traditional naturopathy and herbalism.

The author and her husband live in the Pacific Northwest and value spending time with family including their 10 grandchildren.

Watch for Other books by this author:

Restarting Your Health

To contact us:

educationalresource@tipstoahealthieryou.info

www.ingramcontent.com/pod-product-compliance
Lightning Source LLC
Chambersburg PA
CBHW060519280326
41933CB00014B/3032

* 9 7 8 0 9 8 9 4 7 3 5 4 5 *